Copyright © 20
Coleman Ph.d

All rights reserved. No part of this publication may be reproduced, distributed, or transmitted in any form or by any means, including photocopying, recording, or other electronic or mechanical methods, without the prior written permission of the publisher, except in the case of brief quotation embodied in critical reviews and certian other noncommercial uses permitted by copyright law.

Table of Contents

Introduction 3
What is Healthcare Financing? 7
    Role of finance in Healthcare. 9
Health Care Funding 41
Mode of payment 45
    Private Health insurance 45
    2. Government Insurance Programs 55
    3. Out of pocket 72
Factors That Influence Healthcare Spending Growth 90
Financing Long-Term Care 110
Conclusion 128

Introduction

Health is a basic human right as enshrined in several treaties such as the United Nations Committee on Economic, Social, and Cultural Rights signed by many countries. As a human capital, health determines an individual's economic and job productivity, school-learning capacity, and intellectual growth, which eventually rubs off on the nation. However, prevailing global health inequality necessitated the 2005 World

Health Assembly resolution on Universal Health Coverage (UHC). It recommended that member states should design health financing systems that provide people with access to effective and quality health-care services that do not cause financial hardship on utilization. In pursuance of this objective, goal 3.8 of the Sustainable Development Goals was also designed to achieve UHC (including quality essential service coverage and financial protection for all) after the Millennium Development Goals

(MDGs) ended in 2015. Access to needed health care, plus financial risk protection for all (including the poor and vulnerable groups such as the unemployed, elderly, handicapped, and under-five children)are therefore core principles behind UHC.

Healthcare financing deals with generation, allocation and use of financial resources in the health system. Globally it has become increasingly recognized as an area of major policy relevance to achieve Universal Health Coverage (UHC).

Understanding the country's healthcare financing system allows to recognize current finances available for health, ways to raise more funds for health, mechanisms to efficiently and equitably allocate, purchase and spend finances to improve access to health services and reduce out of pocket expenditures that lead to catastrophe and impoverishment.

What is Healthcare Financing?

Health financing refers to how financial resources are used to ensure that the health system can adequately cover the collective health needs of every person. It is a foundational component that impacts the entire health system's performance, including the delivery and accessibility of primary health care. There are trade-offs inherent within all health financing strategies. For instance, certain payment approaches may enhance quality or access, but also encourage unnecessary use of curative services. Financial resources available for health are always finite, and a government's decisions about resource allocation impact how primary health care is prioritized compared to other components of the health system.

Healthcare involves any medical procedure meant to improve a person's wellbeing. Healthcare financing refers to the management of funds for these medical resources. On a personal level, this type of financing refers to payments regarding hospital care, physician care, dental care, prescriptions, and other personal medical services. When patients cannot pay out-of-pocket medical expenses, healthcare financing works as credit and enables them to receive care.

Role of finance in Healthcare.

Financial management has many objectives, such as:

- Proper mobilization.
- Maintaining proper cash flow.
- Respond to regulations
- Proper utilization of finance.
- Creating reserves.
- Wealth maximization.

1. Diagnosis codes and their impact on reimbursement

Diagnostic coding is the conversion of written details on illnesses, injuries and diseases into codes following a certain classification. Any health care provider, pharmacy, medical equipment supplier or physician filling and submitting a claim to any third party, has to adhere to the set new codes, ICD-10-CM to describe the diagnoses of the patient so as to make the provision of services easier.

As an inclusion in the implementation of the ICD-10, the new DRG grouper practices will be required to transform the new codes into the DRGs to proceed with payment. For the inpatient services, the rates of reimbursement depend on the rates of cases negotiated and this directly impacts the DRGs.

Medical records ought to be coded to determine the revenue neutral and what it means for the health care industry. Health care providers may be limited to interpreting revenue neutrality or lack enough data to evaluate the issue. In another instance updates to the ICD-10 may impact the reimbursement where the payment policies are to be changed as well as the reporting system which will be based on the diagnostic codes.

Based on the current contract reviews, there ought to be a critical evaluation when dealing with provisions that focus on revenue neutrality, policy and manual compliance.

Features of third-party payers

A third party payer is an entity that is contracted with the reimbursement and management of health care expenses. Examples of third-party payers are public insurers, private insurers, self-insurance who cater for the expenses from their own incomes and commercial insurers. This type of insurance is a great income source for health care providers in the health care industry.

The health insurance companies were created by the government so as to help the public against health care burdens. The third party payers cater for the healthcare expenses on behalf of the patients. The patients pay a premium and in other occasions co-pays to these third-party payers and in most instances, they help reduce the finances of the patients. Normally, the third party payers do not pay all the expenses as there are deductibles that are first cleared by the patient.

Reimbursement Methods Used and Effects of Coding On Reimbursement

There are five common methods of hospital reimbursement; shared savings, bundled payments, fee-for-service, value-based reimbursement and discount from billed charges. First, fee-for-service is a model that includes specified negotiated rates for every service of procedure required; nonetheless, overtime and other additional management components and cost controls are encompassed.

Second, a discount from billed charges affords the providers with the lowest level of risk with the payer allowing reimbursement at an agreed discount employing the Charge Description Master which functions by tracking the activity and the billing services.

Third, Value-Based Reimbursement model compensates the health care providers using a fee-for-service technique using quality and resourceful components. Fourth, the shared savings model gives onward incentives and offers lower risks to individuals to enhance harmonization of outcomes and care based on a recognized patient population. Last, bundled payments make available reimbursements to the health care providers for explicit care episodes.

The reimbursement for health care services and procedures is made by commercial payers such as United Health care, Aetna or federal intermediaries that represent health programs. The claims made by the health care providers employing the procedure codes and the medical diagnosis determine the reimbursement.

Medical coding has a significant impact on the performance of the revenue cycle. The health care organizations cannot afford to make mistakes that may impair its operations thus has to use quality medical coding. Quality medical coding is also important to any provider as it saves them from denied claims.

Denial of claims can strain the organization as it is a major strain on the revenue where payments to the providers can be withheld, delayed or stopped. Preferably, combating any instance that may lead to denial is the best option to prevent associated costs and controls. When there is denial, the cost of working them out is not regarded as an expense but an investment that will return high returns.

Regulation does play a vital role in the healthcare industry. It is the responsibility of various governing bodies to protect the public from multiple health dangers and also provide many programs for public health & welfare. It is essential to track and analyze financial ratios in health care organizations. The rations, such as Analyzing debt-to-capitalization ratio, indicates the strength and value of an organization. These ratios also help in managing cash flow and maintaining the long term finances of health care organizations.

2. Revenue Health Care

The Healthcare Financial Management Association defines revenue cycle as "all administrative and clinical functions that contribute to the capture, management, and collection of patient service revenue." Basically, then, the revenue cycle is everything that happens from the moment a patient account is created (at intake, whether that's a doctor's office, outpatient clinic, tertiary care center or other site) through payment for the particular treatment, surgery, or care package.

For the revenue cycle to work most effectively it must be predictable. That means its processes must be executed correctly, which is no small task. An early error can derail the process at multiple points along the way, causing errors in billing, slow payments, and other negative actions. Getting things back on track can be time-consuming and costly.Healthcare revenue cycle management begins when a patient makes his or her appointment to seek medical services and ends when all claims and patient payments have been collected. However, the life of a patient's account is not as straightforward as it seems.

To start, when a patient arranges an appointment, administrative staff must handle the scheduling, insurance eligibility verification, and patient account establishment.

Pre-registration is key to optimizing healthcare revenue cycle management processes. During this step, employees create a patient account that details medical histories and insurance coverages.

Achieving a Healthy Financial Circulatory System

The healthcare revenue cycle can be likened to the body's blood flow—if it's cut off in one spot, the entire system is affected. That's why it's important to look at the different administrative and clinical functions that make up the cycle and ensure that each is properly functioning. Any technical or operational solution should consider:

System Integration: A siloed revenue cycle will lead to lost revenue. Review all integrated software and hardware systems and combine patient electronic health records, accounting, billing, and collections.

Billing and Claims Management: Improve productivity and speed payables by reducing denials and rejected claims through staff training on denial-management processes, better point-of-service collections, and decreased delays in patient billing.

Contact Analysis: A fully fledged data collection and management system, alongside a well thought out strategy, will help providers to negotiate better rates and contracts with payers.

Coding: Physicians and supporting personnel must ensure that they are coding everything correctly, as a single mistake can lead to overbilling and failed audits.

Clinical Documentation: Like coding, all electronic documentation solutions must integrate with other revenue-collection and monitoring procedures to ensure fewer rejected claims.

HOW DOES TECHNOLOGY HELP DRIVE HEALTHCARE REVENUE CYCLE MANAGEMENT?

Health IT and EHR systems have helped to streamline and provide more accuracy to healthcare revenue cycle management strategies. Many organizations use technology to track claims throughout their lifecycles, collect payments, and address claim denials. Ultimately, these technologies facilitate a steady stream of revenue.

Approximately 4,201 hospitals have already invested in healthcare revenue cycle management technologies, which have been especially useful for handling both traditional fee-for-service claims and value-based reimbursement arrangements as the industry transitions to new payment models.

Healthcare revenue cycle management solutions are expected to become even more popular. Investments in healthcare revenue cycle management software and services are predicted to grow by 15.51 percent over the next couple of years. The total spent on revenue cycle management solutions around the world is also projected to reach $7.09 billion by 2020.

Many providers have benefitted from automating common issues with healthcare revenue cycle management, such as payer-improving payer-provider communications, recommending appropriate ICD-10 codes, monitoring medical billing processes, and even scheduling patient appointments.

While these technologies can be expensive, some providers choose to consolidate with other healthcare organizations to invest in healthcare revenue cycle management solutions or outsource some revenue cycle management functions, such as collections.

To adapt to the new healthcare changes and achieve optimal revenue cycle performance, health systems can follow five best practices:

1. Identify and Measure the Right Metrics

The first step to revenue cycle optimization is understanding what to measure. Whether finance teams choose to measure revenue capture or uncollectable accounts, identifying and tracking the right metric is the foundation of short- and long-term success.

The revenue cycle is a complex process full of moving parts, making it difficult to measure every step or handoff throughout the lifecycle of a claim Although it's a tall task, health systems achieve real change when they can measure every handoff throughout the process.

2. Define Clear Lines of Accountability

Precise measurement allows clear lines of accountability. Clear lines of accountability along with clear reporting structures enable leaders to understand who is responsible for which specific metric, and therefore, responsible for driving the performance of that metric.

Identifying and measuring the right metrics also makes the health system accountable to itself. With an accurate baseline of metrics, revenue cycle teams can measure the success of new interventions, make changes accordingly, and report back to leadership, showing accountability for the resources allotted. The ability to quickly measure the effectiveness of new processes is especially helpful in a volatile market when health systems are trying new interventions to grow and improve the patient experience.

3.Create Consistent Workflows

Established, standardized workflows create a uniform, disciplined approach to any process within the revenue cycle. The workflow should look the same throughout the revenue cycle process, no matter the point of access. Ensuring workflows are well-documented and teams are following the workflows correctly are critical components of effective handoffs throughout the revenue cycle journey.

One cohesive, agreed-upon approach also allows revenue cycle leaders to more effectively train staff and help them understand the process at a higher level. Understanding the revenue cycle goals at a high level, and how each person's role fits within the big picture, empowers leaders systemwide to consider the complete revenue cycle in the decision-making process.

4. Define Key Performance Indicators

Revenue cycle leaders need to comprehend that data and metrics don't equate to information. Data and metrics are the building blocks to reach meaningful information, but a crucial in-between step is developing key performance indicators (KPIs). KPIs play a valuable role in helping staff identify the data that will drive decision making.

Leaders should choose KPIs according to relevancy and organizational goals and apply KPIs where they can affect real change. Another essential part of the KPI development phase is developing indicators for each process at the functional level, not just at a high level. KPIs need to target metrics that will help solve problems and drive change within the workflow. KPIs should drive most important organizational decisions, so leaders should review them regularly and choose wisely.

5. Understand the Right Metrics at the Right Place at the Right Time

Leaders can drive real change when they can access the right metrics. For example, a chief financial officer might be more interested in overall strategic metrics instead of operational measures, such as bill edits or late-

...large metrics, but a VP or director-level leader wants to consider more granular, detailed data while making financial decisions. Production measures and overturned denial metrics could be significant operational insights to a manager who can drive change in that area. In this way, establishing the needed metrics for the targeted role means actionable information surfaces to the person who has the power to change it.

Health Care Funding

Who Are Healthcare Providers?

The healthcare provider you're probably the most familiar with is your primary care physician (PCP) or the specialists you see when you need certain specific medical care. But there are all different types of healthcare providers. Any type of healthcare service you might need is provided by some type of healthcare Provider.

Here are some non-physician examples of healthcare providers:

- The physical therapist that helps you to recover from your knee injury
- The home health care company that provides your visiting nurse
- The durable medical equipment company that provides your home oxygen or wheelchair

- Your pharmacy
- The laboratory that draws and processes your blood tests
- The imaging facility that does your mammograms, X-rays, and magnetic resonance imaging (MRI) scans
- The speech therapist that works with you to make sure you can swallow food safely after a stroke
- The outpatient surgery clinic where you had your colonoscopy done

- The specialty laboratory that does your DNA test
- The urgent care center or walk-in clinic in your neighborhood shopping center
- The hospital where you receive inpatient (or in some cases, outpatient) care

Mode of payment

Health care providers (such as doctors and hospitals) are paid by the following:

- Private health insurance
- Government insurance programs
- People themselves (personal, out-of-pocket funds)

Private Health insurance

Private health insurance refers to health insurance plans marketed by the private health insurance industry, as opposed to government-run insurance programs. Private health insurance currently covers a little more than half of the U.S. population.

Private health insurance includes employer-sponsored plans, which cover about half of the American population. Another 6 percent of Americans purchase private coverage outside of the workplace in the individual/family health insurance market, both on and off-exchange.

There are also a variety of types of private health insurance that are much less regulated than regular major medical coverage. This includes short-term health plans, fixed indemnity plans, critical illness plans, accident supplements, dental and vision insurance, etc. These types of coverage are all sold by private health insurance companies, but are generally only suitable to serve as supplemental coverage as opposed to a person's only health coverage (or, in the case of short-term health insurance, to cover a person for a very limited time period).

The Patient Protection and Affordable Care Act (PPACA, or Affordable Care Act [ACA]), which became effective in 2014, is U.S. health care reform legislation intended, among other things, to increase the availability, affordability, and use of health insurance. Many of the ACA's provisions involve an expansion of the private insurance market. It creates incentives for employers to provide health insurance and originally required that nearly all people not covered by their employer or a government insurance program (for example, Medicare or Medicaid) purchase private health insurance (individual mandate). Changes to the ACA ended the individual mandate in 2019.

The ACA requires creation of health insurance exchanges, which are government-regulated, standardized health plans that are administered and sold by private insurance companies. Exchanges may be established within each state, or states may join together to run multistate exchanges. The federal government also may establish exchanges in states that do not do so themselves. There are separate exchanges for individuals and small businesses. The ACA requires that private insurance plans do the following:

- Put no annual or lifetime limits on coverage
- Have no exclusions for preexisting conditions

- Allow children to remain on their parent's health insurance up to age 26
- Provide limited variations in price (premiums can vary based only on age, geographic area, tobacco use, and number of family members)
- Allow for limited out-of-pocket expenses (based on an individual's or family's income)
- Not discontinue coverage (called rescission) except in cases of fraud
- Cover certain defined preventive services with no cost-sharing

- Spend at least 80% to 85% of premiums on medical costs

Recent and impending changes that will affect the ACA include:

Stopping government funding of premium tax credits and cost-sharing reductions

Expansion of association health plans (AHPs) and health reimbursement arrangements (HRAs), which are less expensive and less comprehensive than ACA marketplace plans

Reduced regulatory burden imposed by the Notice of Benefit and Payment Parameters (NBPP), which will give states more leeway in defining essential health benefits

Repeal of the individual mandate

These changes are intended to reduce government and individual spending on health plans, but some authors warn that overall spending on health care may not be reduced and that there may be increased numbers of uninsured or inadequately insured people.

Who gets private health insurance plans?

According to the Kaiser Family Foundation, 49% of Americans get their health insurance through employer-sponsored insurance as a benefit. So if you've ever had insurance through your job, or through someone else's job as a dependent, then you've probably been enrolled in private health insurance.

Private health insurance doesn't have to come from an employer-sponsored group health insurance plan, though. Some people decide to buy individual health insurance directly from health insurance companies, local health insurance brokers, or online health insurance marketplaces

2. Government Insurance Programs

Government health care refers to the federal or state health insurance exchanges, commonly referred to as exchanges, that provide government subsidies to reduce the cost of insurance premiums. It also refers to government programs such as Medicare, Medicaid, TRICARE and VA Health Care.Government provides funds to health care institutions to initiate certain programs that contribute to the betterment of healthcare system. Its primary aim is to cover the cost of health care requirements and basic necessities.

Government Plans were established by the Affordable Care Act to provide every American with quality health coverage that is truly affordable and attainable. There are four types of Government Plans. Known as the "metal plans," they are categorized as. Bronze, Silver and Gold.

State Children's Health Insurance Program: This program was designed to help provide coverage for uninsured children when their family's income was below average but too high to ualify for Medicaid. The federal government provides matching funds to states for health insurance for these families

Children and Youth with Special Health Care Needs: This program coordinates funding and resources to provide care to people with special health needs

Tricare: This program covers about 9 million active duty and retired military personnel and their families (DHA), a component of the Military Health System).

Veterans Health Administration (VHA): This government-operated health care system provides comprehensive health services to eligible military veterans. About 9 million veterans are enrolled

Indian Health Service: This system of government hospitals and clinics provides health services to about 2 million American Indians and Alaskan natives living on or near a reservation (see also Indian Health Service—The Federal Health Program for American Indians and Alaska Natives).

The Federal Employee Health Benefits (FEHB) Program: This program allows private insurers to offer insurance plans within guidelines set by the government, for the benefit of active and retired federal employees and their survivors (see also The Federal Employees Health Benefits (FEHB) Program—U.S. Office of Personnel Management).

Substance Abuse and Mental Health Services Administration (SAMHSA): This agency within the U.S. Department of Health & Human Services leads public health efforts to advance the nation's behavioral health Refugee Health Promotion Program: This program provides short-term health insurance to newly arrived refugees.

History of Government Healthcare

2009 was not the first year that government healthcare was talked about, and Obama was far from the first president to push for it; past presidents had proposed the idea decades before and taken steps in this direction. Democrat Harry Truman, for example, was the first U.S. President to urge

Congress to legislate government healthcare coverage for all Americans.

According to Healthcare Reform in America by Michael Kronenfield, President Franklin Roosevelt intended for Social Security to also incorporate healthcare coverage for seniors, but shied away for fear of alienating the American Medical Association.

In 1965, President Lyndon Johnson signed into law the Medicare program, which is a single-payer, government healthcare plan. After signing the bill, President Johnson issued the first Medicare card to former President Harry Truman.

In 1993, President Bill Clinton appointed his wife, well-versed attorney Hillary Clinton, to head a commission charged with forging a massive reform of U.S. healthcare. After major political missteps by the Clintons and an effective, fear-mongering campaign by Republicans, the Clinton healthcare reform package was dead by Fall 1994. The Clinton administration never tried again to overhaul healthcare, and Republican President George Bush was ideologically opposed to all forms of government-funded social services.

Again in 2008, healthcare reform was a top campaign issue among Democratic presidential candidates. Presidential candidate Barack Obama promised that he would "make available a new national health plan to all Americans, including the self-employed and small businesses, to buy affordable health coverage that is similar to the plan available to members of Congress."

Pros of Government Healthcare

Iconic American consumer advocate Ralph Nader summed up the positives of government-funded healthcare from the patient's perspective:

- Free choice of doctor and hospital;
- No bills, no co-pays, no deductibles;

- No exclusions for pre-existing conditions; you are insured from the day you are born;
- No bankruptcies due to medical bills;
- No deaths due to lack of health insurance;
- Cheaper, Simpler and more affordable;
- Everybody in. Nobody out
- Save taxpayers billions a year in bloated corporate administrative and executive compensation costs.

Other important positives of government-funded healthcare include:

47 millions Americans lacked healthcare insurance coverage as of the 2008 presidential campaign season. Soaring unemployment since then caused the ranks of the uninsured to swell past 50 million in mid-2009. Mercifully, government-funded healthcare provided access to medical services for all uninsured, and lower costs of government healthcare caused insurance coverage to be significantly

more accessible to millions of individuals and businesses.

Doctors and other medical professionals can now focus on patient care and no longer need to spend hundreds of wasted hours annually dealing with insurance companies. Patients, too, no longer need to fritter inordinate amounts of time haggling with insurance companies.

Cons of Government Healthcare

Conservatives and libertarians generally oppose U.S. government healthcare mainly because they don't believe that it's a proper role of government to provide social services to private citizens. Instead, conservatives believe that healthcare coverage should continue to be provided solely by private-sector, for-profit insurance corporations, or possibly by non-profit entities.

In 2009, a handful of Congressional Republicans suggested that perhaps the uninsured could obtain limited medical services via a voucher system and tax credits for low-income families.

Conservatives also contended that lower-cost government healthcare would impose too great of a competitive advantage against for-profit insurers.

The Wall Street Journal argued: "In reality, equal competition between a public plan and private plans would be impossible. The public plan would inexorably crowd out private plans, leading to a single-payer system,".

From the patient's perspective, the negatives of government-funded healthcare include:

- A decrease in flexibility for patients to freely choose from a vast cornucopia of drugs, treatment options, and surgical procedures offered today by higher-priced doctors and hospitals.

- Fewer potential doctors may opt to enter the medical profession due to decreased opportunities for high compensation. Fewer doctors, coupled with skyrocketing demand for doctors, could eventually lead to a shortage of medical professionals and to longer waiting periods for appointments.

3. Out of pocket

When care is not covered by other sources, people pay out of their own funds. They often must use their savings to pay small bills and must borrow (including using credit cards) to pay large bills.

Flexible spending accounts are offered by some employers. Through these accounts, employees can choose to have a limited amount of money deducted from their paychecks to pay for out-of-pocket health care expenses. The money deducted is not subject to federal income taxes. However, the account does not earn interest, and if any money is unused at the end of the year, the employee does not get it back.

Health savings accounts can also be used to pay out-of-pocket expenses. These accounts earn interest, and any unused money is not lost. However, to be eligible to use a health savings account, people must have a health insurance plan that has lower premiums (the fee paid to have insurance) and higher deductibles (the fee paid each time a health service is used) than a traditional health plan. Such plans are called high-deductible health plans.

In the United States, about 17% of health care costs are paid for out-of-pocket. Having to pay for health care out-of-pocket contributes significantly to many bankruptcies in the United States.

Strategies to reduce out-of-pocket payments

In recent years, an increasing number of countries have initiated health financing policy reforms and actions to address concerns over high levels of out-of-pocket payments. Although there is no magic bullet, available information illustrates that countries can succeed with well-designed policies and strategies to reduce OOP and its negative impacts. The main strategies that countries use include to:

- abolish user fees and charges in public health facilities;
- target and exempt specific population groups such as the poor and vulnerable, pregnant women and children from official payments; and

target and exempt a range of health services such as maternal and child care from official payments and deliver them free of charge.

These strategies need political support, decision-making and proper preparation. User fee abolition and exemption can have a large impact on both demand and supply of health services. They likely increase the demand for services which subsequently affects the workload of health workers.

On supply side, they can have drastic impact on the income of public health facilities. Unless substitutive sources for user fee revenues are not found, health service availability, quality, and supply of medical products will suffer and deteriorate.

Pros

1.You Get Unlimited Primary Care Services

There are almost 900 such practices across 48 states and Washington, D.C., according to DPCFrontier.com, a website that provides support and guidance to doctors who are launching DPC practices. That's up from 273 locations in 39 states in 2015. An estimated 500,000 patients are receiving care from DPC practices.

Every DPC practice is different, but typically they offer general medical services such as prevention screenings, wellness visits, and diagnostic tests, as well as minor urgent care services, such as stitches or treatment for a rash.

Given this menu of services, many people using DPCs could ultimately spend less on healthcare compared with a traditional insurance plan if they end up requiring frequent visits.

Three-quarters of those with employer insurance have copays (out-of-pocket fees per office visit) for primary care that average $25, and one-quarter have coinsurance (a fee based on a percentage of cost of a visit), which averages 19 percent, according to the Kaiser Family Foundation. And 81 percent have deductibles that average $1,500 before insurance kicks in.

For those with chronic health problems that need close monitoring, such as diabetes or heart disease, having access to DCP services can be especially cost-effective and convenient. Some practices have dispensaries where you can purchase your prescriptions and offer lab tests such as EKGs on site. Some even make house calls if you're not feeling well enough to get to the doctor's office.

2. Your Doctor Can Really Get to Know You

Even healthier patients may be attracted to the convenience and personal attention you can get in direct primary care. No more booking appointments months in advance, and you can spend more time with your doctor, who can get a better understanding of your medical history.

3. Minimal waiting lists for major procedures

You won't have to wait a long time to see a surgeon or specialist if you're in the United States. In a study conducted by the Commonwealth Fund, it was concluded that 57% of Canadians wait more than 4 weeks to get an appointment with a specialist. In the US, only 23% wait longer than 4 weeks to see a specialist.

Although the medical systems in these two countries often get compared, the truth is that it's much easier to get an appointment or surgery in the United

States. In the US, there is minimal wait time even for complex procedures.

The Cons

1.Health-care services are expensive

The biggest issue Americans have with the current health-care model is that medical services are extremely expensive. In case you don't have insurance or are under-insured, you'll have to pay medical costs out of your pocket. People who don't get insurance also have a very limited number of services they can get access to.

It's worrying that medical debt is the leading cause of bankruptcy in the United States. What a lot of Americans don't realize is that the standard Medicare coverage isn't enough to provide the treatment for certain treatments and procedures.

2.Limited insurance coverage

The majority of Americans get health insurance through their employers. That means that in the event that they lose their job, they can lose their coverage. When someone doesn't have a job, it can be impossible for them to continue paying for insurance. The fact that you could easily lose your healthcare insurance is why most Americans are now in favor of medical system reform.

Lack of transparency

What nearly every medical service available in the US lacks is price transparency. People are not able to shop around and figure out what their most budget-friendly option is. Healthcare is what Americans spend most of their family budget on after housing.

In order for the health-care system in the United States to improve, there needs to be price transparency for medical costs. People simply don't know what to expect when they go to a hospital because the same procedure (even if performed by the same physician) has a different price in each institution.

Today, only 12% of the US population is opposed to price transparency in health care. Meanwhile, hospitals claim that the reason why prices are not transparent is that it allows them to offer discounts to insurance agencies.

Consumer Protections Are Scarce

At least 25 states have passed legislation that generally defines DPC services as being outside the scope of state insurance regulation. This eases the costly regulatory burden for physicians who operate in these practices and enables them to offer low monthly fees. But it also means DPC patients mostly lack the consumer protections mandated by the Affordable Care Act, such as coverage of preexisting conditions and prohibitions against charging more based on gender.

That could be a problem if you should ever have a dispute with your DPC provider over how your care is handled or what services should be covered—perhaps differing definitions of what should be routine care paid by the membership fee. For those with health plans regulated by state insurance departments, you can often get help from these authorities.

Factors That Influence Healthcare Spending Growth

The reasons behind healthcare spending growth are complex and involve a number of interacting factors, according to the Medicare Payment

Advisory Commission. In its annual report to Congress this month, MedPAC identified the following spending trend influencers.

1.Use of expensive new diagnostic tests and treatments

Use of expensive tests and treatments may contribute to increasing health care costs more than any other factor. Use may be appropriate or inappropriate, but in either case, cost is increased.

An example of appropriate but expensive treatment is the use of clot-dissolving (thrombolytic, or fibrinolytic) drugs or a procedure to clear the arteries (such as angioplasty) to treat a heart attack. These treatments are very effective and save lives. But many new and expensive treatments are ineffective, are only slightly better, or are used inappropriately in people who are unlikely to benefit. For example, bones (vertebrae) in the lower back are sometimes fused together to treat chronic low back pain. Many experts think this treatment is ineffective and/or greatly overused.

How often these expensive treatments are used varies greatly from region to region and sometimes from doctor to doctor. For some disorders (such as coronary artery disease), the results of treatment on health are no better in regions where some expensive treatments are used very often than in regions where they are used less often.

2. Technology.

According to MedPAC, technology is credited as having the most significant effect on healthcare spending growth, with studies identifying it as the reason behind anywhere from 38 percent to more than 65 percent of spending growth.

3. Increased costs of health care goods and services

Drug costs have increased. One reason is the increasing cost of developing a new drug, often about $1 billion. Because drug development costs so much, drug companies are not motivated to develop drugs that are less profitable, such as vaccines, drugs used to treat rare disorders, and even antibiotics. This reluctance can negatively affect public health by, for example, limiting the number of drugs and vaccines available to prevent and treat serious infections.

4. Market power.

Provider market power also drives spending growth. Hospitals, physicians and other providers have been consolidating at a rapid rate, and merging with others can give them greater market power over insurers and more leverage in payment rate negotiations, according to MedPAC. Studies have found consolidation can lead to an increase of 5 percent or more in hospital prices.

5. Health insurance coverage.

Getting health insurance coverage can potentially reduce patients' incentives to seek the most efficient, lowest-priced care, according to MedPAC. One study of an insurance coverage experiment in Oregon found people randomly selected for Medicaid coverage used 25 percent more services than an uninsured control group. However, the recent trend of employers and insurers placing more fiscal responsibility on patients' shoulders in the form of higher coinsurance, deductibles and copayments has contributed to slower growth rates recently.

6. Overuse of specialists

Specialists are increasingly providing more care, partly because the number of primary care physicians is decreasing and partly because more and more people want to see a specialist.

Specialty care is often more expensive than primary care. Specialists charge more and may do more tests than primary care doctors. Also, people who have more than one disorder may require several specialists (who have a more narrow focus) to evaluate and treat them, when one primary care doctor (who has a broader focus) might be able to do so.

7.High administrative costs

The percentage of health care dollars spent on administration is estimated to be 20 to more than 30%. Most of these costs come from private insurance companies; however, the Affordable Care Act now limits the amount that private insurance can spend on administrative costs. Companies that provide private insurance spend money on marketing and evaluation of applicants to identify those with preexisting disorders or the potential for developing a disorder. These processes do not improve health care. Also, having to deal with many different private insurance plans typically increases administrative costs for health care providers by making processes (such as claim submission and coding) more complicated and time-consuming.

8. Doctor fees

Doctors in the United States are paid more than many other professionals in this country and more than doctors in many other countries. Part of the reason is that doctors in other countries typically spend far less on their medical education and malpractice insurance than those in the United States do, and the costs of running an office in other countries are lower.

Doctor fees account for about 20% of total health care costs. Thus even a significant reduction in these fees would have only a modest effect on overall costs.

9.Malpractice costs

These costs include

Malpractice insurance

Tests and procedures done to protect against being sued for malpractice, rather than to ensure the health of the person (called defensive medicine)

Doctors, other health care providers, health care institutions, and drug and device manufacturers pay premiums for malpractice insurance. These premiums cover claim settlements and the overhead and profits of malpractice insurance company. Ultimately, these costs, at least in part, are passed on to the government and/or consumers.

These costs and the threat of lawsuits can be burdensome for individual doctors (particularly those in certain high-risk specialties and geographic areas). Nonetheless, the amount of money spent on premiums (the fee paid to an insurance company to have malpractice insurance) each year is only about 0.3% of total health care costs. Also, the amount of money spent in malpractice settlements represents an even smaller percentage of health care costs. Thus, even a major reduction in malpractice settlements would not lower total health care costs substantially, although it could greatly benefit some doctors.

10. Defensive medicine

Defensive medicine refers to tests or treatments done to protect doctors and other health care providers from being sued for malpractice. These tests and treatments may not be medically justifiable based on the person's situation. For example, a doctor may hospitalize a person even though the person could probably be effectively treated as an outpatient.

How much defensive medicine actually costs is difficult to measure. Few well-designed studies of costs have been done, and estimates from these studies vary greatly. Costs are hard to determine partly because defensive medicine is defined subjectively. That is, it is based on the doctor's judgment about whether doing a test or treatment is needed. Doctors can vary substantially and legitimately when making such a decision about a specific person's situation. Only a relatively few situations have clear and specific guidelines for testing.

Even when defensive testing is identified, determining how much money could be saved is complicated. Decreasing the amount of defensive testing involves comparing the actual costs of care with and without an extra test or treatment. These costs differ from how much people are charged and from what they are reimbursed for.

Also, whether laws to limit compensation to people suing for malpractice lowers health care costs is unclear.

11. Aging of the population

Although often cited as a factor (about one third of overall health care costs occur in the last year of life), the aging population is probably not responsible for recent increases in costs because many of the baby boomers have not yet reached old age. Also, more effective health care is tending to delay serious illness in older people. However, costs may be affected more as the baby boomers age. The proportion of the population over 65 is predicted to increase from about 15% in 2016 to almost 20% after 2030.

12. Demographics and patient characteristics.

Changes in the age and health status of the population can make a significant difference in healthcare spending; the

CBO has identified the aging baby boomer population as a major driver of spending growth. Additionally, national income growth and expanding insurance coverage leads to investment and changes in health technologies, according to MedPAC.

Financing Long-Term Care

Nearly eleven million people in the United States use some form of long-term care, and that number is projected to double by 2050. Persons age eighty-five and over are the fastest growing segment of the population in most developed countries; they tend to be less healthy and are more likely to have chronic conditions that require care than younger cohorts.

1 While there is some evidence that disability rates among older people have declined in recent decades,

2 this trend may be reversing.

3 The total number of older people is rising, and the number of years of care that people with disabling conditions

require may also be increasing. All this translates into a greater demand for long-term care services in the years ahead.4 Although health insurance may cover medical care needed by people living with chronic illness, it provides little if any coverage for personal care services like bathing, dressing, preparing meals, getting out of bed, and using the toilet.

The aging population, and the increased incidence of chronic illness, also places greater pressure on family caregivers to provide these services.

This development affects women disproportionately as they tend to adopt most of the responsibility for the care of older parents and spouses, regardless of whether these women participate in the labor force. In fact, research indicates that women who are in the labor force are just as likely to act as caregivers as women who are not.5 Along with the economic burden, caregiving can also lead to health problems for the caregivers themselves. Many studies have found that stress, less time spent with family/friends, amount of medication use, lost time at work, misuse of alcohol or prescription drugs, incidence of coronary heart disease, and depression are all associated with caregiving.

In addition to these effects on unpaid caregivers, the growing demand for long-term care is placing increasing strain on public budgets. Medicaid, America's federal-state health insurance program for people with low incomes, is the largest source of funds for long-term care. For decades, people have hoped that the purchase of private long-term care insurance might help to address these concerns, but the demand for private products remain extraordinarily low, and the supply of them is actually shrinking.

Generally, health plans do not cover long term care. Health insurance usually provides medical care for health conditions or illness for a shorter period of time, but please check with your health plan and ask what your plan covers.

You should also know that Medicare or disability only covers certain types of care. Many believe Medicaid is another option, but this requires you to spend all of your own funds before you are eligible. Basically, some choose to impoverish themselves, but in the process give up freedom to choose where and how they receive long term care.

who pays for long term care?

Health insurance and Medicare only pay for long term care in certain situations. Health insurance usually provides medical care for health conditions or illness for a shorter duration. Long term care may not always involve medical treatment, but require assistance with daily activities over a longer period of time.

Here are some ways to cover the costs of long term care. Be sure to click on the Contact tab and sign up for the booklet on long term care options, so that you can make informed and be better prepared.

Personal income and savings

Health savings accounts

Home equity options

Life insurance options

Long term care insurance

Public long term care insurance program.

Challenges in Financing Long-Term Care

Inadequate Coverage at Unfavorable Prices

On a more immediate and concrete level, the prices and policies of private insurance companies also discourage most people from purchasing long-term care insurance. The only way long-term care insurance could be financially viable is for people to purchase coverage when they are young adults. If people wait until they are much older, there is a serious problem of adverse selection, because insurance companies do not want to sell policies to people who are likely to need care only a few years after they start paying premiums.

Most of the time, insurance companies simply refuse to sell policies to older individuals in poor health, but even if they agree to sell an older person insurance, the price is likely to be so high that it would not make sense to purchase it. Under this structure, the only way to make long-term care insurance premiums affordable is to enroll people when they are younger—long before they are likely to need assistance. But from the perspective of insurance companies, this is still a problem. Even if you could overcome the factors that limit demand for this insurance among younger people, insurance companies are still unlikely to offer an attractive product, because it is difficult to predict the costs of long-term care decades into the future.

To cope with this uncertainty, insurance companies use two strategies. First, they tend to set high rates to guard against significant increases in the cost of future care. Second, they often set a cap on policy benefits based on the current costs of long-term care services. For example, a typical plan would not only place a cap on the total dollar amount available to pay for nursing home or home- and community-based services, it would also limit the number of years it would cover care (often to no more than three years of coverage). The high premiums make the product unaffordable to a large part of the market. At the same time, the benefit caps make the product less attractive to potential buyers. For example, one study estimates that the load of a "typical" policy purchased at age sixty-five in 2010 is 32 cents on the dollar. It is also much greater for men (55 cents) than for women (13 cents).

Because these traditional long-term care insurance plans are unattractive to insurance companies and potential buyers, insurance companies have recently tried to market combined life and long-term care insurance products. These products allow policy holders to use the benefits to pay for long-term care, rather than cash payments after death; but if policy holders do not need long-term care, they are able to bequeath the cash benefits to others. As with the traditional policies, however, the benefits are often capped at levels that are much lower than the average cost of long-term care, so it seems unlikely to significantly address the problem.

LTSS is an insurable risk, yet sales of private LTCI policies have faltered. Because neither the government nor individuals alone can meet all demands for LTSS financing, middle-income Americans should have a functional, sustainable private LTCI marketplace to help them pay for LTSS should they need it. If policymakers take action to stabilize the LTCI market and make it accessible to more Americans, those in need of LTSS will be able to extend the time they remain at home or in community-based settings.

For the roughly half of Americans aged 65 and over who willexperience a high level of LTSS need, establish a lower-cost,limited-benefit private LTCI product, called "retirement LTCI,"which would also be more sustainable for carriers than traditional products

This lower-cost product would be designed to cover two to fouryears of benefits after a cash deductible or waiting period is met.

The product would also include coinsurance.To make these policies more affordable and to encourageAmericans to plan for LTSS need while they save for retirement,employees may use funds in retirement accounts to pay retirement LTCI premiums (early withdrawals would be penalty-free).

To efficiently expand coverage, recommendations include providing incentives for employers to offer retirement LTCI on an opt-out basis through workplace retirement plans and permitting the sale of retirement LTCI through state and federal insurance marketplaces.

Conclusion

As healthcare financing moves away from a fee-for-service model toward innovative payment models, including capitation, a healthcare system's success will rest on its ability to proactively manage the health of its patient population. Coordinating with other local stakeholders by creating a pediatric care network is an effective way to address population health. Clear guidelines or regulations are needed for the implementation and the coordination between payers, providers and insurers. Finally, a comprehensive benefit package should be offered for the insurance to be attractive and maximize the financial protection.

Made in the USA
Coppell, TX
21 January 2022